Your Mediterranean Cookbook

Super-Easy and Tasty Recipes to Enjoy Mediterranean Diet and Avoid Bad Habits

I0145872

America Best Recipes

© **Copyright 2020 - All rights reserved.**
The content contained within this book may not be reproduced, duplicated or transmitted without direct written permission from the author or the publisher.
Under no circumstances will any blame or legal responsibility be held against the publisher, or author, for any damages, reparation, or monetary loss due to the information contained within this book. Either directly or indirectly.

Legal Notice:
This book is copyright protected. This book is only for personal use. You cannot amend, distribute, sell, use, quote or paraphrase any part, or the content within this book, without the consent of the author or publisher.

Disclaimer Notice:
Please note the information contained within this document is for educational and entertainment purposes only. All effort has been executed to present accurate, up to date, and reliable, complete information. No warranties of any kind are declared or implied. Readers acknowledge that the author is not engaging in the rendering of legal, financial, medical or professional advice. The content within this book has been derived from various sources. Please consult a licensed professional before attempting any techniques outlined in this book.
By reading this document, the reader agrees that under no circumstances is the author responsible for any losses, direct or indirect, which are incurred as a result of the use of information contained within this document, including, but not limited to, — errors, omissions, or inaccuracies.

Table of contents

Dill Tapas

Preparation Time: 5 minutes

Cooking Time: 0 minutes

Servings: 8

Ingredients:

- ½ tsp. garlic powder
- 2 cups plain yogurt
- ½ cup dill, chopped
- ¼ tsp. ground black pepper
- 2 pecans, chopped
- 2 tbsp. lemon juice

Directions:

1. Put all ingredients in the bowl and stir well with the help of the spoon.

Nutrition: 77 Calories, 4.5g Protein, 6.7g Carbs, 3.4g Fat, 0.8g Fiber

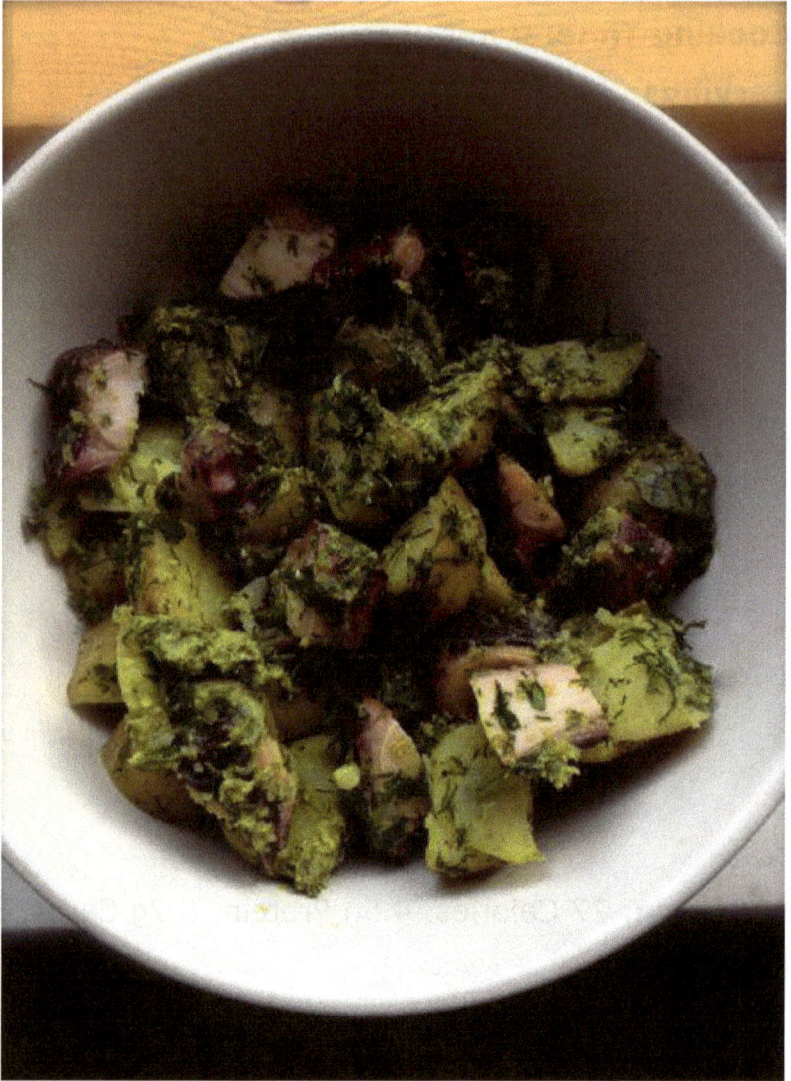

Sour Cream Dip

Preparation Time: 10 minutes

Cooking Time: 0 minutes

Servings: 8

Ingredients:

- 4 oz yogurt
- ¼ tsp. chili flakes
- ¼ tsp. salt
- 2 avocados, peeled, pitted
- 1 tsp. olive oil
- ½ tsp. lemon juice
- 2 tbsp. fresh parsley, chopped

Directions:

1. Put all ingredients in the blender and blend until smooth.
2. Store the dip in the closed vessel in the fridge for up to 5 days.

Nutrition: 138 Calories, 1.4g Protein, 5g Carbs, 13.4g Fat, 3.4g Fiber

Arugla Antipasti

Preparation Time: 5 minutes

Cooking Time: 0 minutes

Servings: 8

Ingredients:

- 2 oz chives, chopped
- 1 cup arugula, chopped
- 2 cups chickpeas, canned
- 1 jalapeno pepper, chopped
- 1 tbsp. avocado oil
- 1 tsp. lemon juice

Directions:

1. Put all ingredients in the bowl and stir well.

Nutrition: 188 Calories, 10g Protein, 30.9g Carbs, 3.3g Fat, 9.1g Fiber

Goat Cheese Dip

Preparation Time: 10 minutes

Cooking Time: 8 minutes

Servings: 4

Ingredients:

- 3 oz goats cheese, soft
- 2 oz plain yogurt
- 2 oz chives, chopped
- 1 tbsp. lemon juice
- ¼ tsp. ground black pepper
- 2 bell peppers

Directions:

1. Grill the bell peppers for 3-4 minutes per side.
2. Then peel the peppers and remove seeds.
3. Then put bell peppers in the blender.
4. Add all remaining ingredients, blend them well and transfer in the ramekins.

Nutrition: 92 Calories, 5.9g Protein, 6.5g Carbs, 4.9g Fat, 1.2g Fiber

Mozzarella Dip

Preparation Time: 10 minutes

Cooking Time: 20 minutes

Servings: 10

Ingredients:

- 1-lb. artichoke hearts, diced
- ¾ cup spinach, chopped
- 1 cup mozzarella cheese, grated
- 1 tsp. Italian seasonings
- ½ tsp. garlic powder
- ¼ cup organic almond milk

Directions:

1. Put all ingredients in the saucepan, stir well, and close the lid.
2. Saute the meal on low heat for 20 minutes. Stir it from time to time.
3. Then chill the dip well.

Nutrition: 46 Calories, 2.5g Protein, 5.4g Carbs, 2.2g Fat, 2.6g Fiber

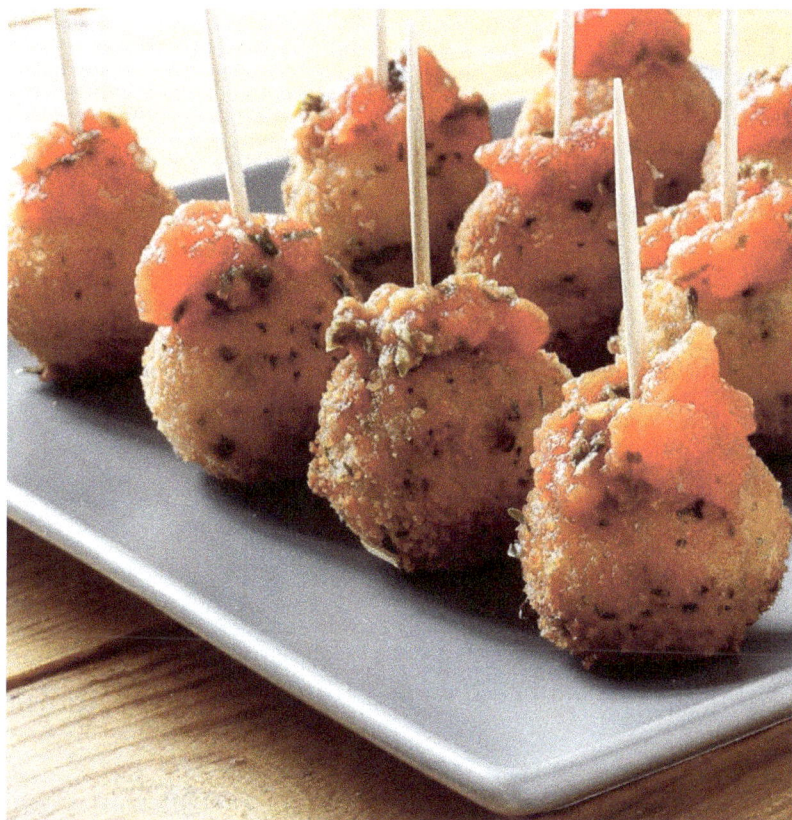

Spicy Salsa

Preparation Time: 40 minutes

Cooking Time: 0 minutes

Servings: 16

Ingredients:

- 3 cups tomatoes, chopped
- 1 tsp. salt
- 1 tsp. white pepper
- ½ cup red onion, chopped
- 1 cup fresh cilantro, chopped
- 1 jalapeno pepper, chopped
- 1 tbsp. olive oil
- 1 tbsp. apple cider vinegar

Directions:

1. Put all ingredients in the salad bowl and mix well.
2. Leave the cooked salsa for 30 minutes in the fridge.

Nutrition: 16 Calories, 0.4g Protein, 1.8g Carbs, 1g Fat, 0.6g Fiber

Cheese Spread

Preparation Time: 10 minutes

Cooking Time: 8 minutes

Servings: 6

Ingredients:

- ½ cup cream cheese
- 1 pickle, grated
- 1 oz fresh dill, chopped
- ¼ tsp. ground paprika

Directions:

1. Carefully mix cream cheese with dill and ground paprika.
2. Then add a grated pickle and gently mix the spread.

Nutrition: 81 Calories, 2.5g Protein, 3.4g Carbs, 7g Fat, 0.8g Fiber

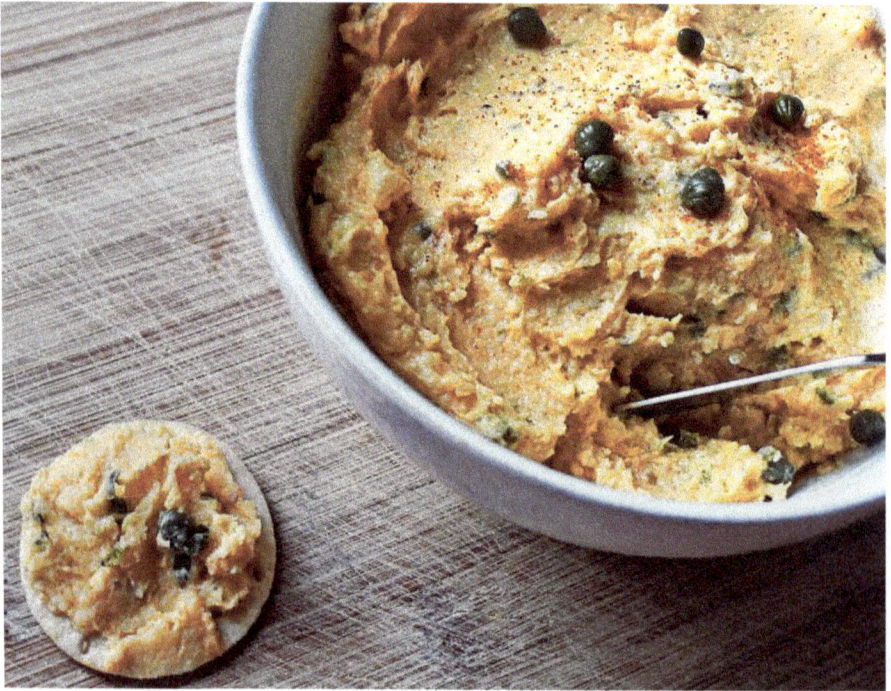

Prosciutto Beans

Preparation Time: 10 minutes

Cooking Time: 0 minutes

Servings: 8

Ingredients:

- 2 cups canned cannellini beans, drained
- 1 tbsp. scallions, diced
- 3 tbsp. olive oil
- ¼ tsp. chili flakes
- 1 tbsp. lemon juice
- 3 oz beef, chopped, cooked

Directions:

1. Put all ingredients in the bowl and stir well.

Nutrition: 219 Calories, 14.1g Protein, 27.7g Carbs, 6.3g Fat, 11.5g Fiber

Carrot Chips

Preparation Time: 5 minutes

Cooking Time: 10 minutes

Servings: 6

Ingredients:

- 2 carrots, thinly sliced
- 1 tsp. salt
- 1 tsp. olive oil

Directions:

1. Line the baking tray with baking paper.
2. Then arrange the sliced carrot in one layer.
3. Sprinkle the vegetables with olive oil and salt.
4. Bake the carrot chips for 10 minutes or until the vegetables are crunchy.

Nutrition: 15 Calories, 0.2g Protein, 2g Carbs, 0.8g Fat, 0.5g Fiber

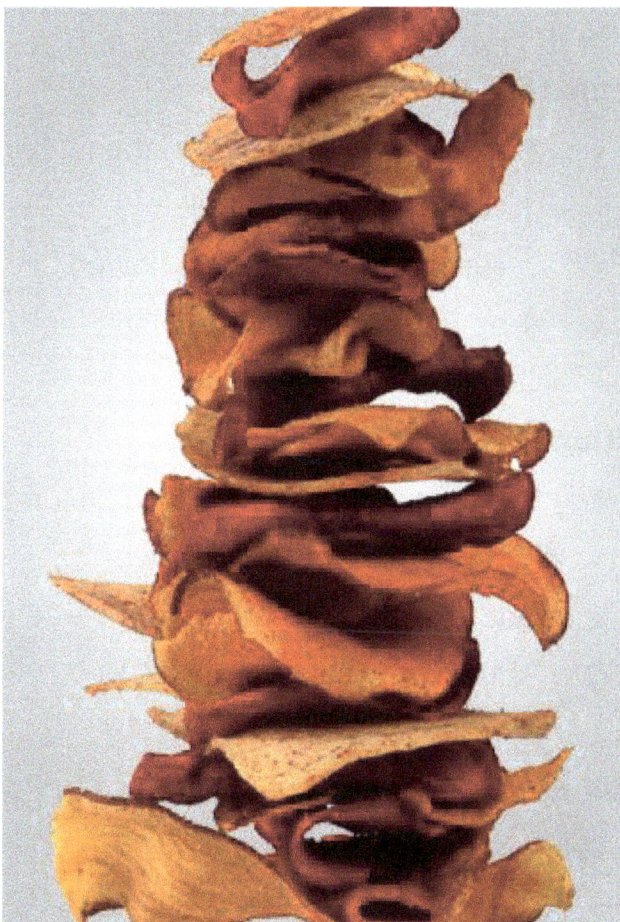

Antipasti Salad

Preparation Time: 10 minutes

Cooking Time: 0 minutes

Servings: 4

Ingredients:

- ½ cup green olives, pitted and sliced
- 1 cucumber, spiralized
- 1 cup cherry tomatoes, halved
- 4 oz Feta cheese, crumbled
- 2 tbsp. olive oil

Directions:

1. Put green olives, spiralized cucumber, and cherry tomatoes in the bowl.
2. Add olive oil and stir well.
3. Then top the salad with Feta.

Nutrition: 185 Calories, 4.9g Protein, 6.9g Carbs, 16.3g Fat, 0.9g Fiber

Black Olives Spread

Preparation Time: 10 minutes

Cooking Time: 0 minutes

Servings: 10

Ingredients:

- 3 cups black olives, pitted
- ½ cup chickpeas, canned
- 1 tsp. Italian seasonings
- 3 tbsp. sunflower oil
- ½ tsp. ground black pepper

Directions:

1. Put all ingredients in the blender and blend until smooth.

Nutrition: 122 Calories,2.3g Protein, 8.7g Carbs, 9.3g Fat, 3.1g Fiber

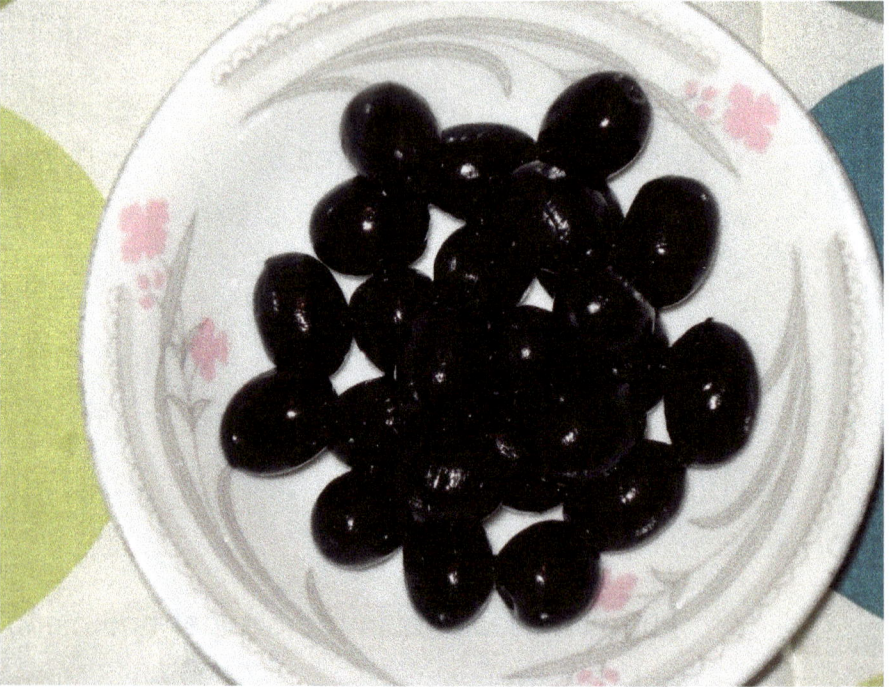

Bell Pepper Antipasti

Preparation Time: 10 minutes

Cooking Time: 4 minutes

Servings: 6

Ingredients:

- 5 bell peppers
- 1 tbsp. olive oil
- 3 tbsp. avocado oil
- ½ tsp. salt
- 2 garlic cloves, minced
- 3 tbsp. fresh cilantro, chopped

Directions:

1. Pierce the bell peppers with the help of a knife and sprinkle with olive oil.
2. Grill the vegetables at 400F for 2 minutes per side.
3. Then peel them and remove seeds.
4. Put the grilled bell peppers in the blender and add all remaining ingredients.
5. Blend the mixture well.

Nutrition: 63 Calories, 1.2g Protein, 8.2g Carbs, 3.5g Fat, 1.7g Fiber

Hummus Rings

Preparation Time: 10 minutes

Cooking Time: 0 minutes

Servings: 4

Ingredients:

- ½ cup hummus
- 2 cucumbers

Directions:

1. Roughly slice the cucumbers and remove the cucumber flesh.
2. Then fill every cucumber ring with hummus.

Nutrition: 74 Calories, 3.5g Protein, 9.9g Carbs, 3.2g Fat, 2.6g Fiber

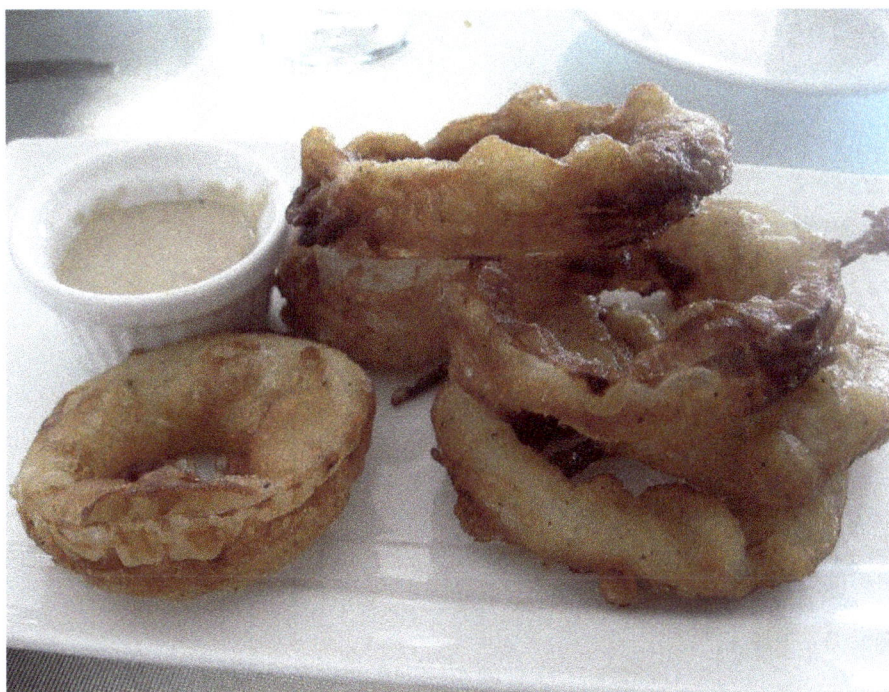

Fish Strips

Preparation Time: 10 minutes

Cooking Time: 0 minutes

Servings: 4

Ingredients:

- 1 cucumber, sliced
- 1 tsp. apple cider vinegar
- 2 tbsp. plain yogurt
- 1 tsp. dried dill
- 3 oz salmon, smoked, sliced

Directions:

1. Arrange the sliced cucumber in the plate in one layer.
2. Then sprinkle them with apple cider vinegar, plain yogurt, and dried dill.
3. Then top the cucumbers with sliced salmon.

Nutrition: 35 Calories, 4.6g Protein, 0.8g Carbs, 1.4g Fat, 0.1g Fiber

Vegetable Balls

Preparation Time: 10 minutes

Cooking Time: 5 minutes

Servings: 8

Ingredients:

- 2 eggplants, grilled
- 2 tbsp. olive oil
- 1 garlic clove, minced
- 1 egg, beaten
- ½ cup oatmeal, ground
- ½ tsp. ground black pepper
- 2 oz Parmesan, grated

Directions:

1. Blend the eggplants until smooth.
2. Then mix up blended eggplants with garlic, egg, oatmeal, ground black pepper, and Parmesan.
3. Make the small balls.
4. Heat the skillet with olive oil and put the eggplant balls inside.
5. Roast them for on high heat for 1 minute per side.

Nutrition: 115 Calories, 5g Protein, 12g Carbs, 6.2g Fat, 5.4g Fiber

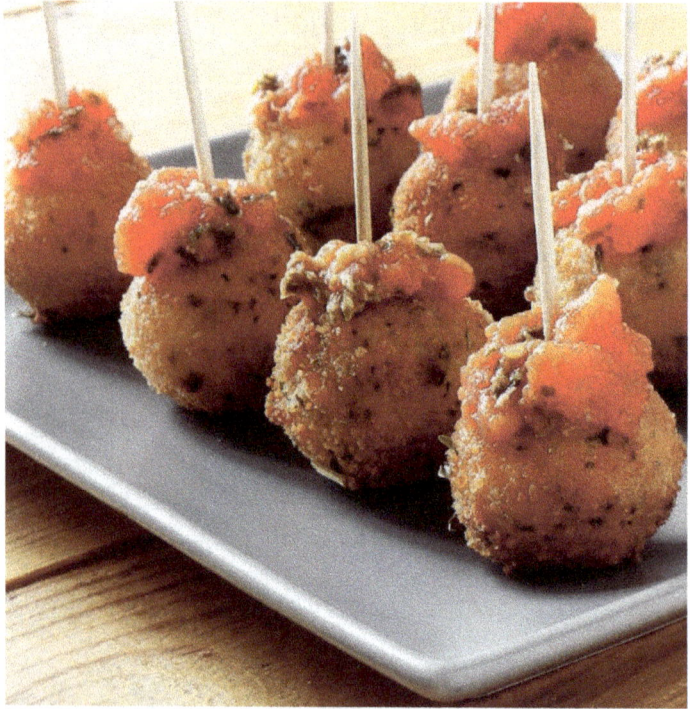

Italian Style Eggplant Chips

Preparation Time: 10 minutes

Cooking Time: 5 minutes

Servings: 10

Ingredients:

- 2 eggplants, thinly sliced
- 1 tsp. ground black pepper
- 1 tsp. Italian seasonings
- 1 tbsp. olive oil

Directions:

1. Rub the eggplant sliced with ground black pepper and Italian seasonings.
2. Then sprinkle the vegetable sliced with olive oil.
3. Grill the eggplant sliced for 2 minutes per side at 400F or until the vegetables are crunchy.

Nutrition: 41 Calories, 1.1g Protein, 6.6g Carbs, 1.8g Fat, 3.9g Fiber

Lentil Dip

Preparation Time: 10 minutes

Cooking Time: 0 minutes

Servings: 7

Ingredients:

- 1 cup green lentils, cooked
- 1 tbsp. apple cider vinegar
- 1 tomato, chopped
- 1 tsp. olive oil
- 2 oz Parmesan, grated

Directions:

1. Mix up all ingredients in the bowl and blend gently with the help of the immersion blender.

Nutrition: 131 Calories, 9.8g Protein, 17.1g Carbs, 2.7g Fat, 8.5g Fiber

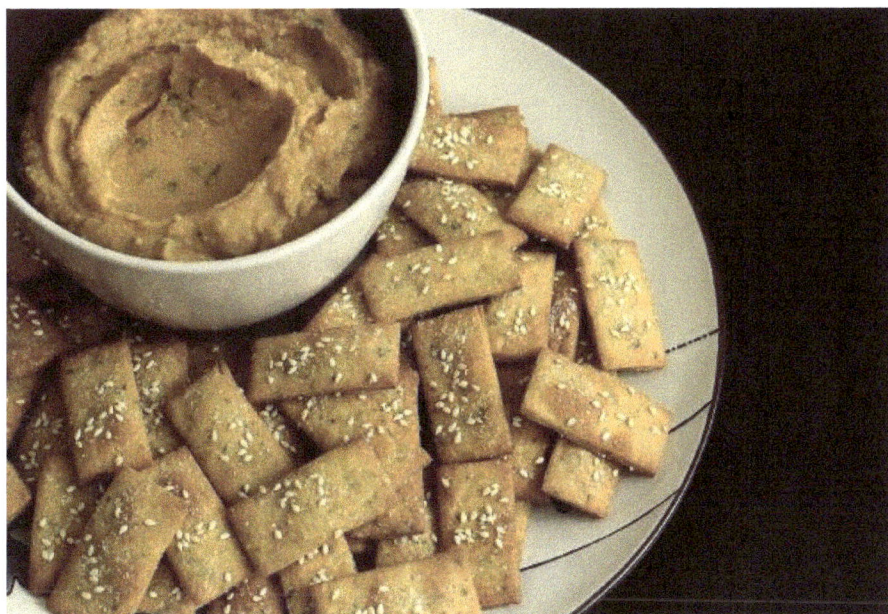

Cheese Baby Potatoes

Preparation Time: 10 minutes

Cooking Time: 20 minutes

Servings: 2

Ingredients:

- 4 baby potatoes
- 2 oz Cheddar cheese, shredded
- ¼ tsp. garlic powder
- 1 tsp. avocado oil

Directions:

1. Cut the baby potatoes into halves and sprinkle with garlic powder and avocado oil.
2. Bake the potatoes for 10 minutes at 365F.
3. Then top them with Cheddar cheese and bake for 10 minutes more.

Nutrition: 136 Calories, 7.7g Protein, 4.5g Carbs, 9.7g Fat, 0.4g Fiber

Tuna Paste

Preparation Time: 5 minutes

Cooking Time: 0 minutes

Servings: 6

Ingredients:

- 7 oz tuna, canned
- 2 tbsp. cream cheese
- 1 tbsp. chives, chopped

Directions:

1. Put all ingredients in the bowl and stir well with the help of the fork.

Nutrition: 73 Calories, 9g Protein, 0.1g Carbs, 3.8g Fat, 0g Fiber

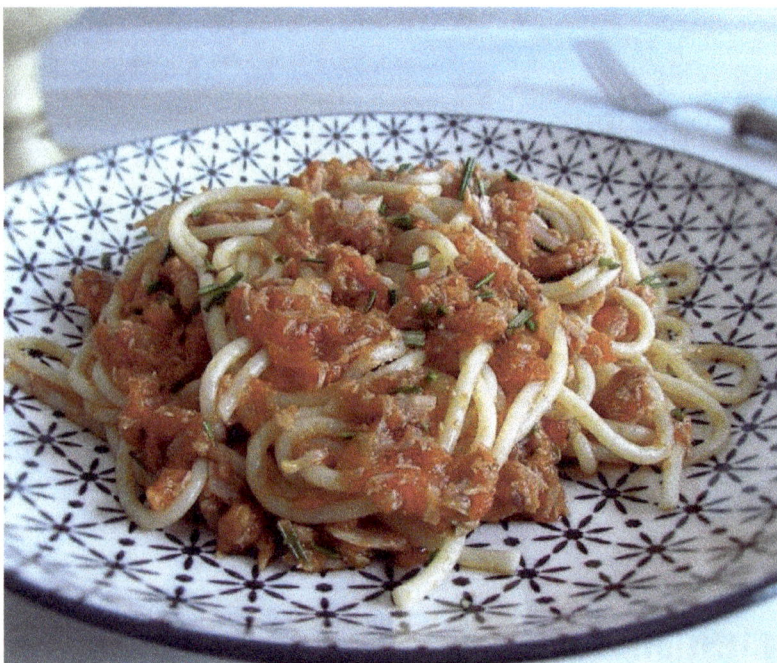

Zucchini Chips

Preparation Time: 5 minutes

Cooking Time: 12 minutes

Servings: 10

Ingredients:

- 2 zucchinis, thinly sliced
- 1 oz Parmesan, grated

Directions:

1. Line the baking tray with baking paper.
2. Put the zucchini in the tray in one layer and top with Parmesan.
3. Bake the chips for 12 minutes at 375F.

Nutrition: 15 Calories, 1.4g Protein, 1.4g Carbs, 0.7g Fat, 0.4g Fiber

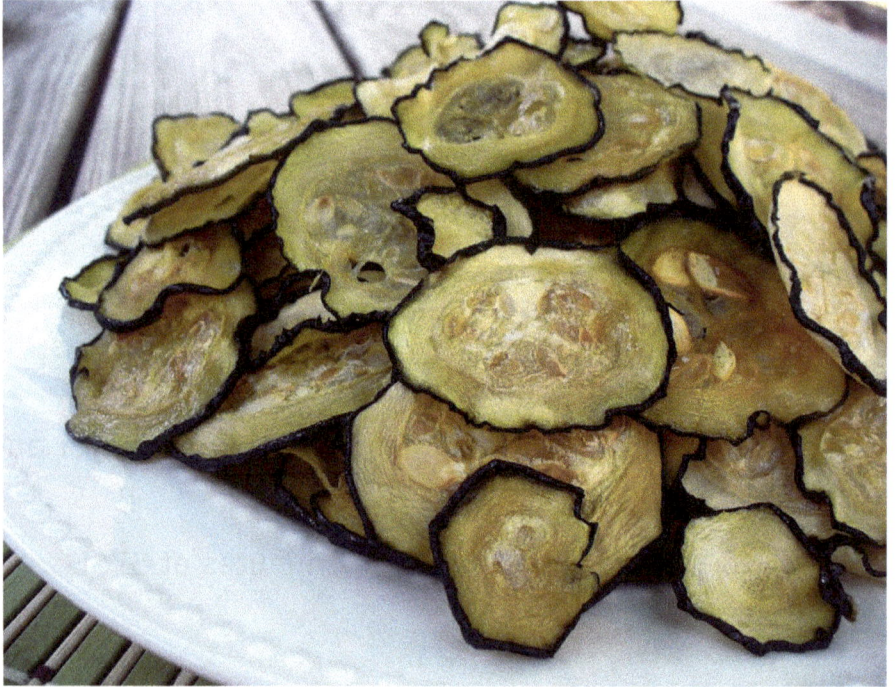

Crunchy Chickpeas

Preparation Time: 5 minutes

Cooking Time: 10 minutes

Servings: 2

Ingredients:

- ¼ cup chickpeas, canned
- 1 tbsp. avocado oil
- 1 tsp. ground paprika

Directions:

1. Line the baking tray with baking paper.
2. Mix up chickpeas with ground paprika and avocado oil and transfer the mixture in the tray. Flatten it gently.
3. Bake the chickpeas for 10 minutes at 400F. Stir them every 2 minutes.

Nutrition: 103 Calories, 5.1g Protein, 16.1g Carbs, 2.5g Fat, 5.1g Fiber

Stuffed Dates

Preparation Time: 5 minutes

Cooking Time: 0 minutes

Servings: 4

Ingredients:

- 4 dates, pitted
- 4 walnuts

Directions:

1. Fill the dates with walnuts.

Nutrition: 75 Calories, 1.5g Protein, 7g Carbs, 5g Fat, 1.4g Fiber

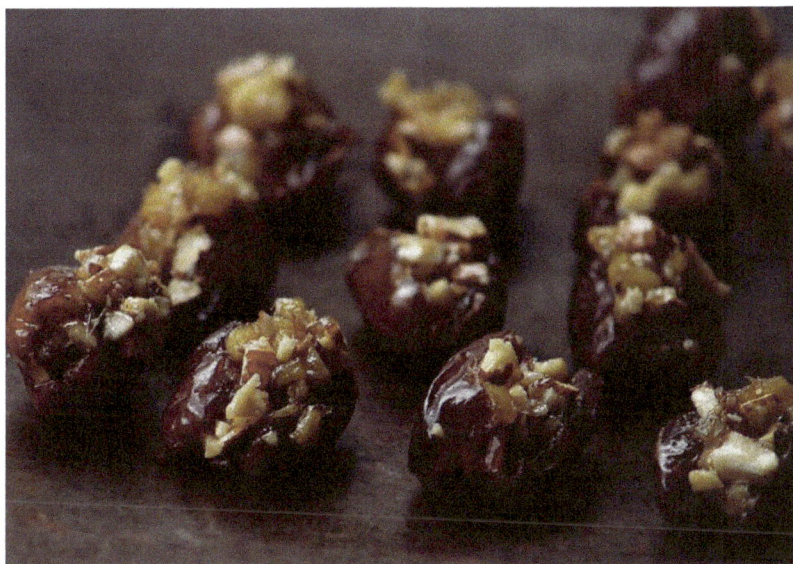

Almond Gazpacho

Preparation Time: 15 minutes

Cooking Time: 0 minutes

Servings: 4

Ingredients:

- ½ cup almonds
- 1 cup cucumbers, chopped
- ½ tsp. minced garlic
- 3 oz water, warm
- 2 oz chives, chopped
- 1 tbsp. sunflower oil
- ¼ cup fresh dill, chopped
- ¼ cup plain yogurt

Directions:

1. Put all ingredients in the blender and blend until smooth.
2. Cool the cooked gazpacho in the fridge for 10-15 minutes.

Nutrition: 127 Calories, 4.6g Protein, 7g Carbs, 9.9g Fat, 2.4g Fiber

Turkey Chowder

Preparation Time: 5 minutes

Cooking Time: 20 minutes

Servings: 2

Ingredients:

- ½ cup ground turkey
- ¼ cup leek, chopped
- 1 tsp. dried rosemary
- 1 cup of water
- 1 cup plain yogurt
- 1 tsp. olive oil

Directions:

1. Roast the ground turkey with olive oil in the pan for 10 minutes. Stir well.
2. Then add all remaining ingredients and close the lid.
3. Cook the chowder for 10 minutes more on the medium heat.

Nutrition: 277 Calories, 29.8g Protein, 10.6g Carbs, 13g Fat, 0.5g Fiber

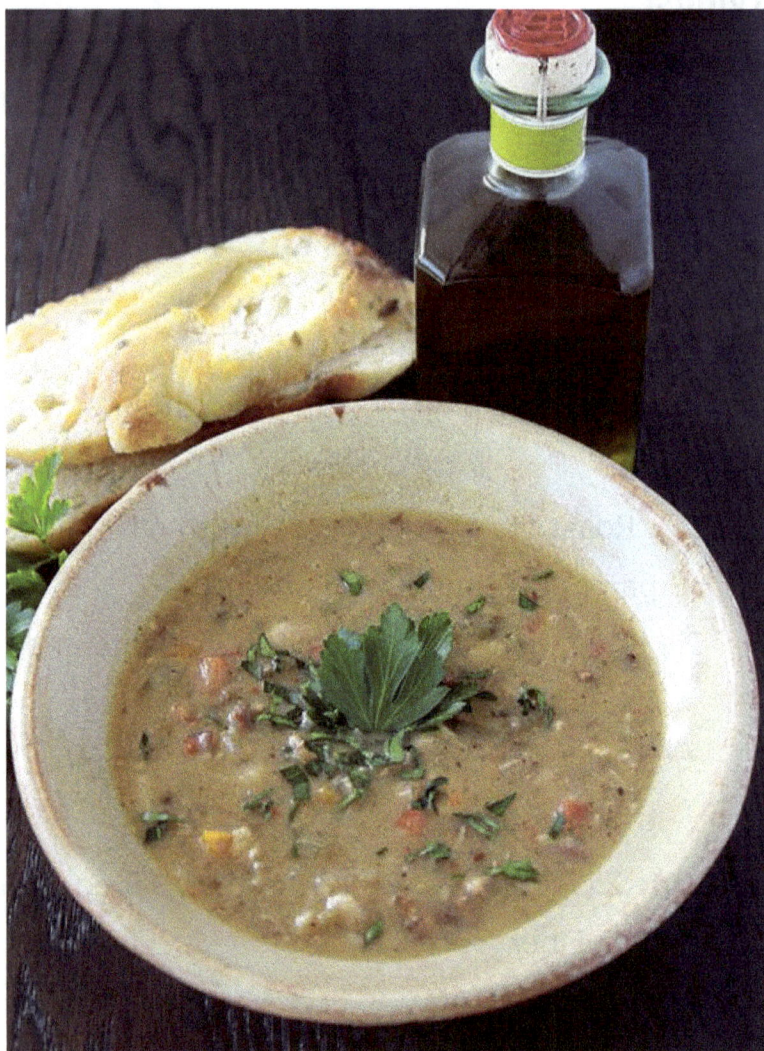

Herb-Topped Focaccia

Preparation Time: 20 minutes

Cooking Time: 2 hours

Servings: 10

Ingredients:

- 1 tbsp. dried rosemary or 3 tbsp. minced fresh rosemary
- 1 tbsp. dried thyme or 3 tbsp. minced fresh thyme leaves
- ½ cup extra-virgin olive oil
- 1 tsp. sugar
- 1 cup warm water
- 1 (¼-oz.) packet active dry yeast
- 2½ cups flour, divided
- 1 tsp. salt

Directions:

1. In a small bowl, combine the rosemary and thyme with the olive oil.
2. In a large bowl, whisk together the sugar, water, and yeast. Let stand for 5 minutes.
3. Add 1 cup of flour, half of the olive oil mixture, and the salt to the mixture in the large bowl. Stir to combine.

4. Add the remaining 1½ cups flour to the large bowl. Using your hands, combine dough until it starts to pull away from the sides of the bowl.

5. Put the dough on a floured board or countertop and knead 10 to 12 times. Place the dough in a well-oiled bowl and cover with plastic wrap. Put it in a warm, dry space for 1 hour.

6. Oil a 9-by-13-inch baking pan. Turn the dough onto the baking pan, and using your hands gently push the dough out to fit the pan.

7. Using your fingers, make dimples into the dough. Evenly pour the remaining half of the olive oil mixture over the dough. Let the dough rise for another 30 minutes.

8. Preheat the oven to 450°F. Place the dough into the oven and let cook for 18 to 20 minutes, until you see it turn a golden brown.

Nutrition:

Calories: 53;

Protein: 12.3g;

Carbs: 3.4g;

Fat: 6.3g

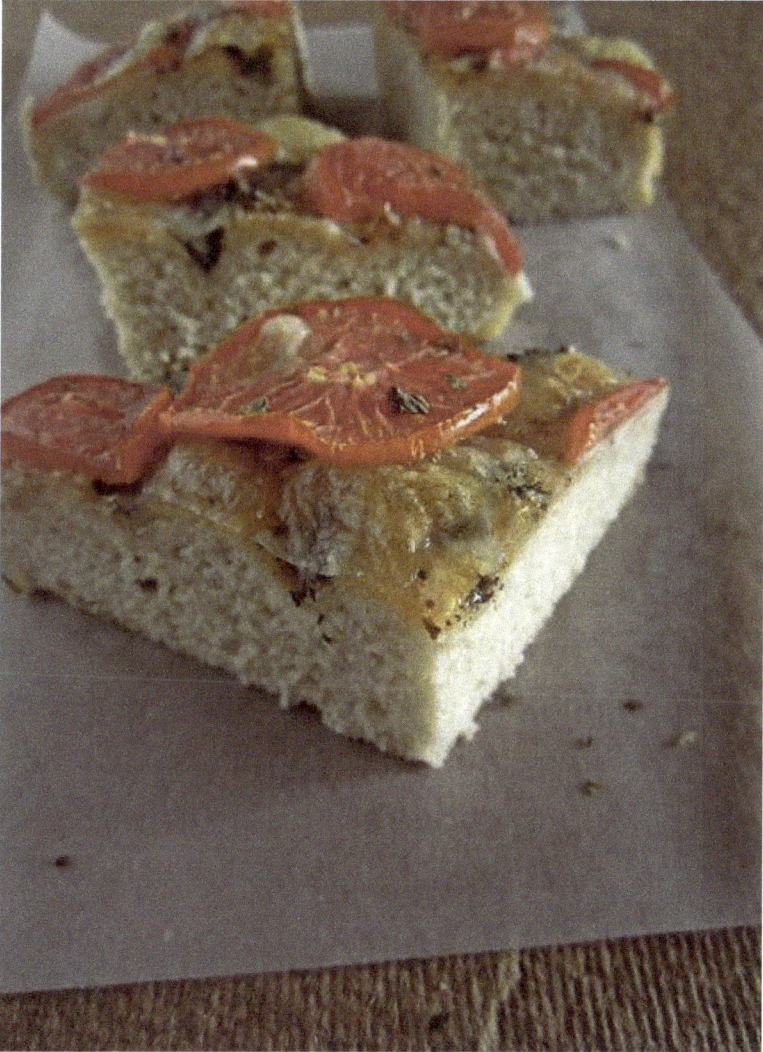

Caramelized Onion Flatbread with Arugula

Preparation Time: 10 minutes

Cooking Time: 25 minutes

Servings: 4

Ingredients:

- 4 tbsp. extra-virgin olive oil, divided
- 2 large onions, sliced into ¼-inch-thick slices
- 1 tsp. salt, divided
- 1 sheet puff pastry
- 1 (5-oz.) package goat cheese
- 8 oz. arugula
- ½ tsp. freshly ground black pepper

Directions:

1. Preheat the oven to 400°F.
2. In a large skillet over medium heat, cook 3 tbsp. olive oil, the onions, and ½ tsp. of salt, stirring, for 10 to 12 minutes, until the onions are translucent and golden brown.
3. To assemble, line a baking sheet with parchment paper. Lay the puff pastry flat on the parchment paper. Prick the middle of the puff pastry all over with a fork, leaving a ½-inch border.

4. Evenly distribute the onions on the pastry, leaving the border.
5. Crumble the goat cheese over the onions. Put the pastry in the oven to bake for 10 to 12 minutes, or until you see the border become golden brown.
6. Remove the pastry from the oven, set aside. In a medium bowl, add the arugula, remaining 1 tbsp. of olive oil, remaining ½ tsp. of salt, and ½ tsp. black pepper; toss to evenly dress the arugula.
7. Cut the pastry into even squares. Top the pastry with dressed arugula and serve.

Nutrition:

Calories: 63;

Protein: 12.3g;

Carbs: 3.4g;

Fat: 6.3g

Quick Shrimp Fettuccine

Preparation Time: 10 minutes

Cooking Time: 10 minutes

Servings: 4

Ingredients:

- 8 oz. fettuccine pasta
- ¼ cup extra-virgin olive oil
- 3 tbsp. garlic, minced
- 1 lb. large shrimp (21-25), peeled and deveined
- 1/3 cup lemon juice
- 1 tbsp. lemon zest
- ½ tsp. salt
- ½ tsp. freshly ground black pepper

Directions:

1. Bring a large pot of salted water to a boil. Add the fettuccine and cook for 8 minutes.
2. In a large saucepan over medium heat, cook the olive oil and garlic for 1 minute.

3. Add the shrimp to the saucepan and cook for 3 minutes on each side. Remove the shrimp from the pan and set aside.
4. Add the lemon juice and lemon zest to the saucepan, along with the salt and pepper.
5. Reserve ½ cup of the pasta water and drain the pasta.
6. Add the pasta water to the saucepan with the lemon juice and zest and stir everything together. Add the pasta and toss together to evenly coat the pasta. Transfer the pasta to a serving dish and top with the cooked shrimp. Serve warm.

Nutrition:

Calories: 83;

Protein: 12.3g;

Carbs: 3.4g;

Fat: 6.3g

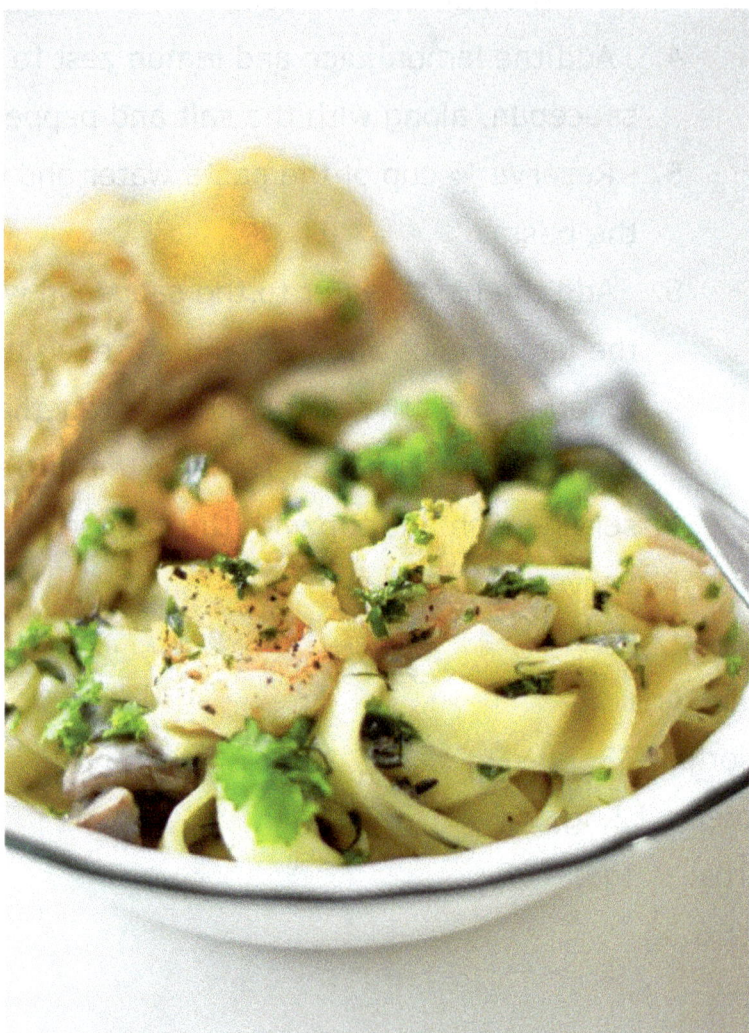

Simple Pesto Pasta

Preparation Time: 10 minutes

Cooking Time: 10 minutes

Servings: 4

Ingredients:

- 1 lb. spaghetti
- 4 cups fresh basil leaves, stems removed
- 3 cloves garlic
- 1 tsp. salt
- ½ tsp. freshly ground black pepper
- ¼ cup lemon juice
- ½ cup pine nuts, toasted
- ½ cup grated Parmesan cheese
- 1 cup extra-virgin olive oil

Directions:

1. Bring a large pot of salted water to a boil. Add the spaghetti to the pot and cook for 8 minutes.
2. Put basil, garlic, salt, pepper, lemon juice, pine nuts, and Parmesan cheese in a food

processor bowl with chopping blade and purée.

3. While the processor is running, slowly drizzle the olive oil through the top opening. Process until all the olive oil has been added.

4. Reserve ½ cup of the pasta water. Drain the pasta and put it into a bowl. Immediately add the pesto and pasta water to the pasta and toss everything together. Serve warm.

Nutrition:

Calories: 113;

Protein: 12.3g;

Carbs: 3.4g;

Fat: 6.3g

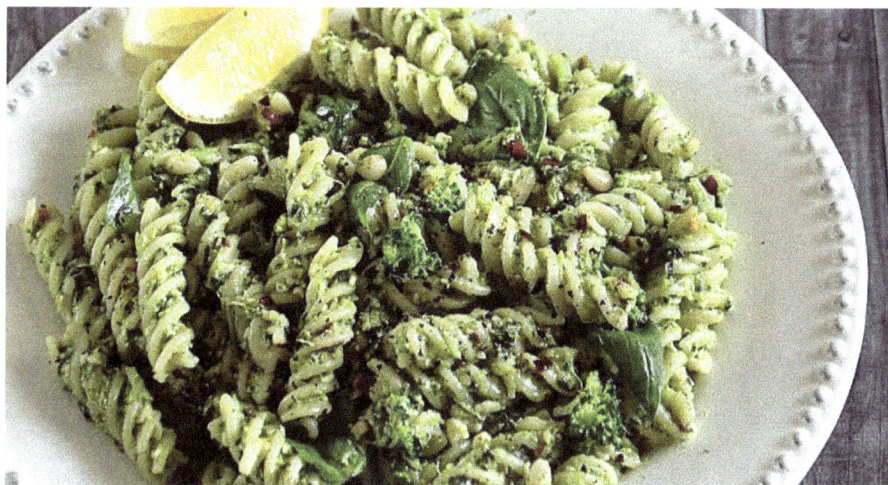

Flat Meat Pies

Preparation Time: 20 minutes

Cooking Time: 15 minutes

Servings: 4

Ingredients:

- ½ lb. ground beef
- 1 small onion, finely chopped
- 1 medium tomato, finely diced and strained
- ½ tsp. salt
- ½ tsp. freshly ground black pepper
- 2 sheets puff pastry

Directions:

1. Preheat the oven to 400°F.
2. In a medium bowl, combine the beef, onion, tomato, salt, and pepper. Set aside.
3. Line 2 baking sheets with parchment paper. Cut the puff pastry dough into 4-inch squares and lay them flat on the baking sheets.

4. Scoop about 2 tbsp. of beef mixture onto each piece of dough. Spread the meat on the dough, leaving a ½-inch edge on each side.
5. Put the meat pies in the oven and bake for 12 to 15 minutes until edges are golden brown.

Nutrition:

Calories: 53;

Protein: 12.3g;

Carbs: 3.4g;

Fat: 6.3g

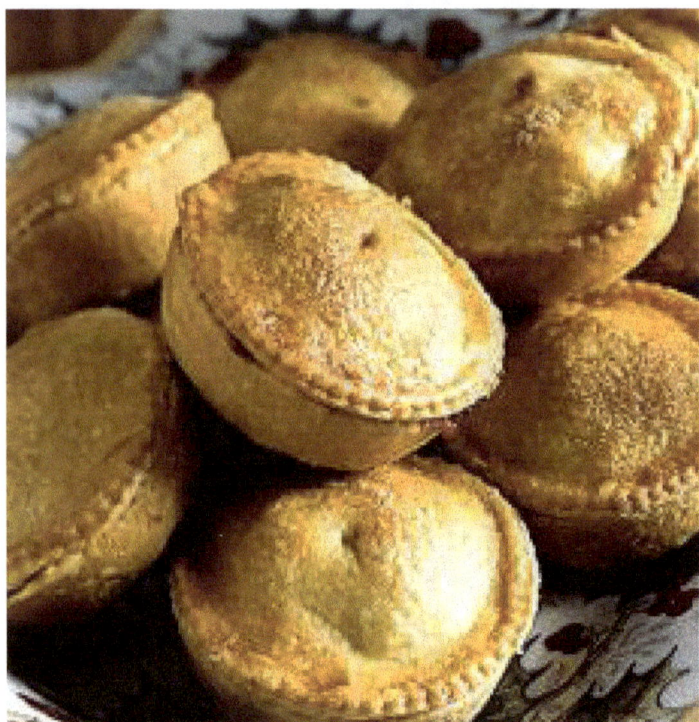

Meaty Baked Penne

Preparation Time: 10 minutes

Cooking Time: 40 minutes

Servings: 6

Ingredients:

- 1 lb. penne pasta
- 1 lb. ground beef
- 1 tsp. salt
- 1 (25-oz.) jar marinara sauce
- 1 (1-lb.) bag baby spinach, washed
- 3 cups shredded mozzarella cheese, divided

Directions:

1. Bring a large pot of salted water to a boil, add the penne, and cook for 7 minutes. Reserve 2 cups of e pasta water and drain the pasta.
2. Preheat the oven to 350°F.
3. In a large saucepan over medium heat, cook the ground beef and salt. Brown the ground beef for about 5 minutes.

4. Stir in marinara sauce, and 2 cups of pasta water. Let simmer for 5 minutes.

5. Add a handful of spinach at a time into the sauce, and cook for another 3 minutes.

6. To assemble, in a 9-by-13-inch baking dish, add the pasta and pour the pasta sauce over it. Stir in 1½ cups of the mozzarella cheese. Cover the dish with foil and bake for 20 minutes.

7. After 20 minutes, remove the foil, top with the rest of the mozzarella, and bake for another 10 minutes. Serve warm.

Nutrition:

Calories: 173;

Protein: 12.3g;

Carbs: 3.4g;

Fat: 6.3g

Mediterranean Pasta with Tomato Sauce and Vegetables

Preparation Time: 15 minutes

Cooking Time: 25 minutes

Servings: 8

Ingredients:

- 8 oz. linguine or spaghetti, cooked
- 1 tsp. garlic powder
- 1 (28 oz.) can whole peeled tomatoes, drained and sliced
- 1 tbsp. olive oil
- 1 (8 oz.) can tomato sauce
- ½ tsp. Italian seasoning
- 8 oz. mushrooms, sliced
- 8 oz. yellow squash, sliced
- 8 oz. zucchini, sliced
- ½ tsp. sugar
- ½ cup grated Parmesan cheese

Directions:

1. In a medium saucepan, mix tomato sauce, tomatoes, sugar, Italian seasoning, and garlic

powder. Bring to boil on medium heat. Reduce heat to low. Cover and simmer for 20 minutes.

2. In a large skillet, heat olive oil on medium-high heat.

3. Add squash, mushrooms, and zucchini. Cook, stirring, for 4 minutes or until tender-crisp.

4. Stir vegetables into the tomato sauce.

5. Place pasta in a serving bowl.

6. Spoon vegetable mixture over pasta and toss to coat.

7. Top with grated Parmesan cheese.

Nutrition:

Calories: 154

Protein: 6 g

Fat: 2 g

Carbs: 28 g

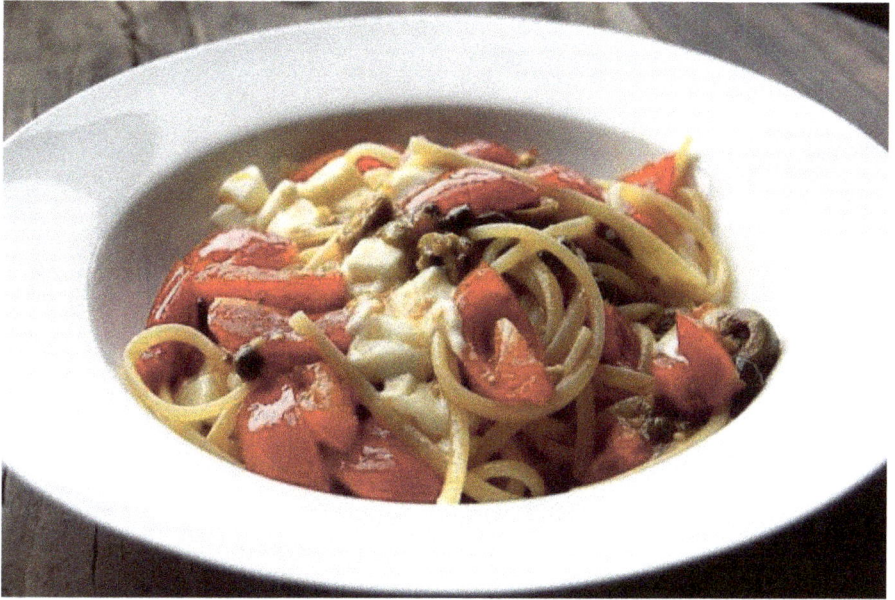

Very Vegan Patras Pasta

Preparation Time: 5 minutes

Cooking Time: 10 minutes

Servings: 6

Ingredients:

- 4-quarts salted water
- 10-oz. gluten-free and whole-grain pasta
- 5-cloves garlic, minced
- 1-cup hummus
- Salt and pepper
- 1/3-cup water
- ½-cup walnuts
- ½-cup olives
- 2-tbsp dried cranberries (optional)

Directions:

1. Bring the salted water to a boil for cooking the pasta.

2. In the meantime, prepare for the hummus sauce. Combine the garlic, hummus, salt, and pepper with water in a mixing bowl. Add the

walnuts, olive, and dried cranberries, if
desired. Set aside.

3.   Add the pasta in the boiling water. Cook the
pasta following the manufacturer's
specifications until attaining an al dente
texture. Drain the pasta.

4.   Transfer the pasta to a large serving bowl
and combine with the sauce.

Nutrition:

Calories: 329

Protein: 12 g

Fat: 13 g

Carbs: 43 g

Cheesy Spaghetti with Pine Nuts

Preparation Time: 10 minutes

Cooking Time: 10 minutes

Servings: 4

Ingredients:

- 8 oz. spaghetti
- 4 tbsp. (½ stick) unsalted butter
- 1 tsp. freshly ground black pepper
- ½ cup pine nuts
- 1 cup fresh grated Parmesan cheese, divided

Directions:

1. Bring a large pot of salted water to a boil. Add the pasta and cook for 8 minutes.
2. In a large saucepan over medium heat, combine the butter, black pepper, and pine nuts. Cook for 2 to 3 minutes or until the pine nuts are lightly toasted.
3. Reserve ½ cup of the pasta water. Drain the pasta and put it into the pan with the pine nuts.

4.   Add ¾ cup of Parmesan cheese and the reserved pasta water to the pasta and toss everything together to evenly coat the pasta.

5.   To serve, put the pasta in a serving dish and top with the remaining ¼ cup of Parmesan cheese.

Nutrition:

Calories: 238;

Protein: 12.3g;

Carbs: 3.4g;

Fat: 6.3g

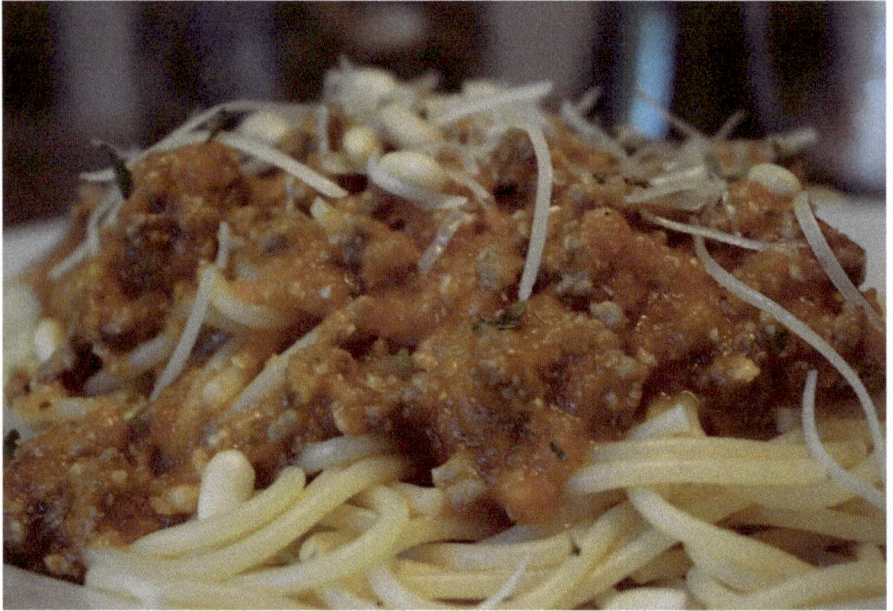

Creamy Garlic-Parmesan Chicken Pasta

Preparation Time: 5 minutes

Cooking Time: 25 minutes

Servings: 6

Ingredients:

- 2 boneless, skinless chicken breasts
- 3 tbsp. extra-virgin olive oil
- 1½ tsp. salt
- 1 large onion, thinly sliced
- 3 tbsp. garlic, minced
- 1 lb. fettuccine pasta
- 1 cup heavy (whipping) cream
- ¾ cup freshly grated Parmesan cheese, divided
- ½ tsp. freshly ground black pepper

Directions:

1. Bring a large pot of salted water to a simmer.
2. Cut the chicken into thin strips.
3. In a large skillet over medium heat, cook the olive oil and chicken for 3 minutes.
4. Next add the salt, onion, and garlic to the pan with the chicken. Cook for 7 minutes.

5. Bring the pot of salted water to a boil and add the pasta, then let it cook for 7 minutes.

6. While the pasta is cooking, add the cream, ½ cup of Parmesan cheese, and black pepper to the chicken; simmer for 3 minutes.

7. Reserve ½ cup of the pasta water. Drain the pasta and add it to the chicken cream sauce.

8. Add the reserved pasta water to the pasta and toss together. Let simmer for 2 minutes. Top with the remaining ¼ cup Parmesan cheese and serve warm.

Nutrition:

Calories: 153;

Protein: 12.3g;

Carbs: 3.4g;

Fat: 6.3g

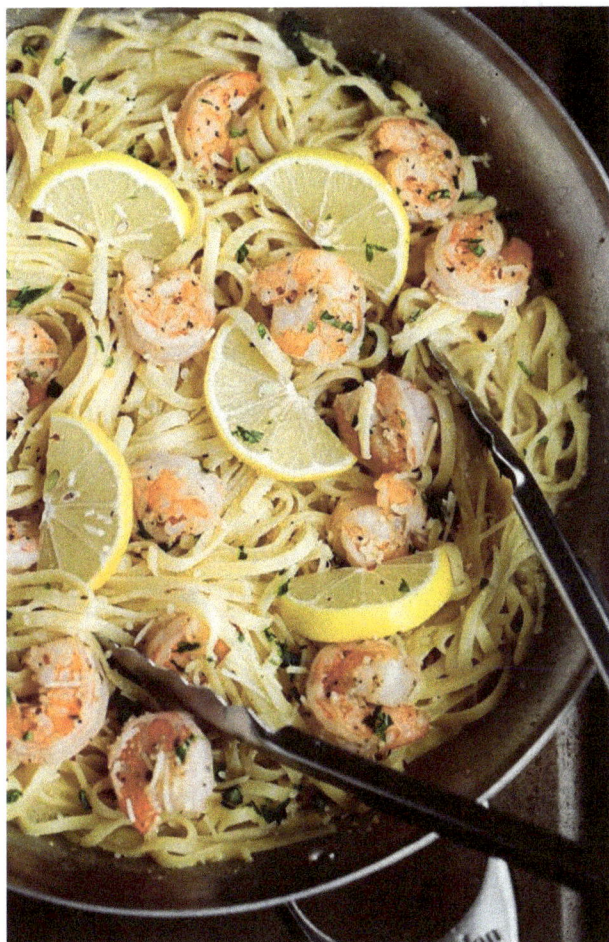

Artichoke Chicken Pasta

Preparation Time: 20 minutes

Cooking Time: 5 minutes

Servings: 4

Ingredients:

- 2 cloves garlic, crushed
- 2 lemons, wedged
- 2 tbsp. lemon juice
- 14 oz. artichoke hearts, chopped
- 1-lb. chicken breast fillet, diced
- ½ cup feta cheese, crumbled
- 1 tbsp. olive oil
- 16 oz. whole-wheat (gluten-free) pasta of your choice
- 3 tbsp. parsley, chopped
- ½ cup red onion, chopped
- 2 tsp. oregano
- 1 tomato, chopped
- Ground black pepper and salt, to taste

Directions:

1. Pour the water into a deep saucepan and boil it. Add the pasta and some salt; cook it as per

package directions. Drain the water and set aside the pasta.

2.   Over medium stove flame, heat the oil in a skillet or saucepan (preferably of medium size).

3.   Sauté the onions and garlic until softened and translucent, stir in between.

4.   Add the chicken and cook until it is no longer pink.

5.   Mix in the tomatoes, artichoke hearts, parsley, feta cheese, oregano, lemon juice and the cooked pasta.

6.   Combine well and cook for 3-4 minutes, stirring frequently.

7.   Season with black pepper and salt. Garnish with lemon wedges and serve warm.

Nutrition: Calories – 486|Fat – 10g|Carbs – 42g|Fiber – 9g|Protein – 37g

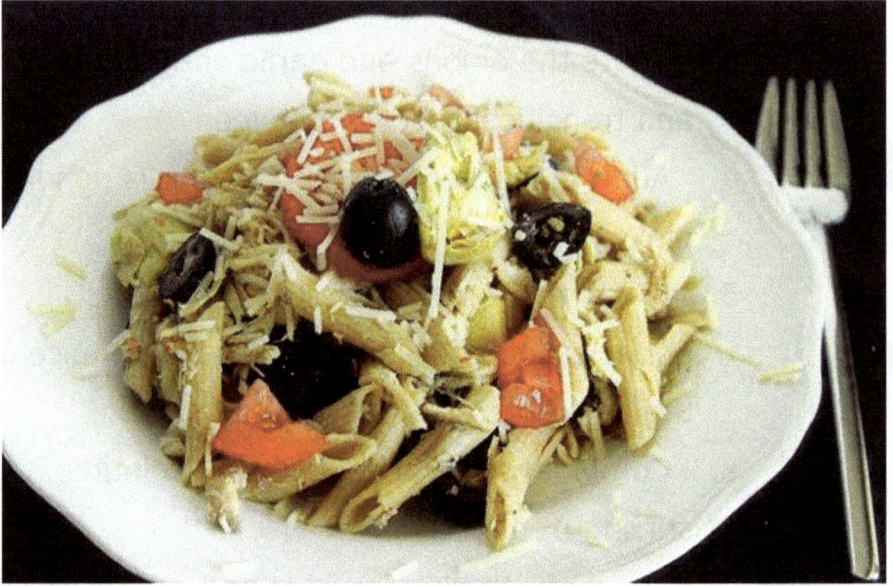

Spinach Beef Pasta

Preparation Time: 30 minutes

Cooking Time: 10 minutes

Servings: 4

Ingredients:

- 1 ¼ cups uncooked orzo pasta
- ¾ cup baby spinach
- 2 tbsp. olive oil
- 1 ½ lb. beef tenderloin
- ¾ cup feta cheese
- 2 quarts water
- 1 cup cherry tomatoes, halved
- ¼ tsp. salt

Directions:

1. Rub the meat with pepper and cut into small cubes.

2. Over medium stove flame; heat the oil in a deep saucepan (preferably of medium size).
3. Add and stir-fry the meat until it is evenly brown.
4. Add the water and boil the mixture; stir in the orzo and salt.
5. Cook the mixture for 7-8 minutes. Add the spinach and cook until it wilts.
6. Add the tomatoes and cheese; combine and serve warm.

Nutrition: Calories – 334 |Fat – 13g|Carbs – 36g|Fiber – 6g|Protein – 16g

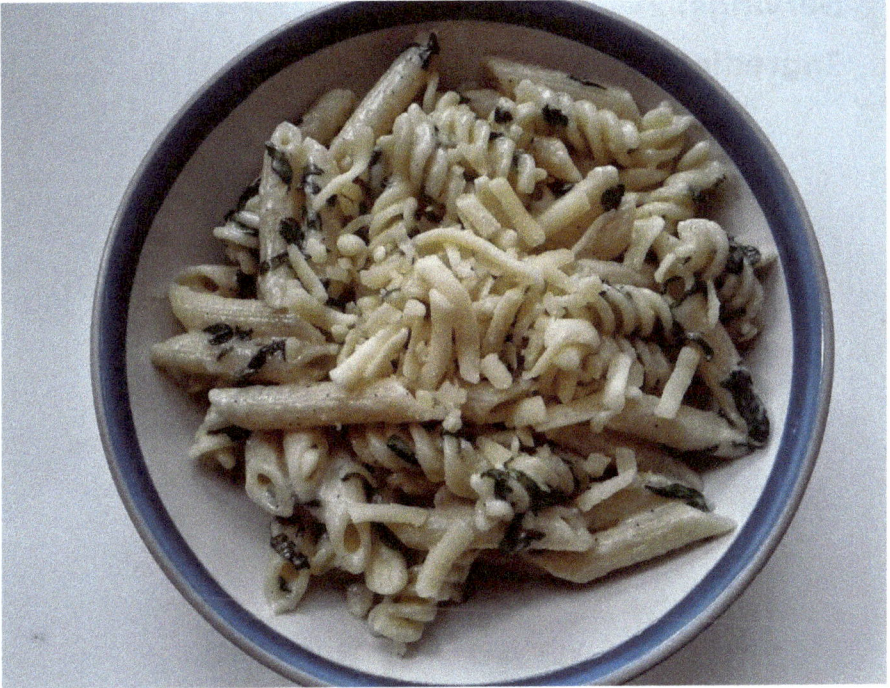

Asparagus Parmesan Pasta

Preparation Time: 25 minutes

Cooking Time: 4 minutes

Servings: 2

Ingredients:

- 1 tsp. extra-virgin olive oil
- 1 tsp. lemon juice
- ¾ cup whole milk
- ½ bunch asparagus, trimmed and cut into small pieces
- ½ cup parmesan cheese, grated
- 2 tbsp. garlic, minced
- 2 tbsp. almond flour
- 2 tsp. whole grain mustard
- 4 oz. whole-wheat penne pasta
- 1 tsp. tarragon, minced
- Ground black pepper and salt, to taste

Directions:

1. Pour the water into a deep saucepan and boil it. Add the pasta and some salt; cook it as per package directions. Drain the water and set aside the pasta.

2. Take another pan, pour 8 cups of water and let it come to boiling. Add the asparagus and boil until it is soft. Drain and set aside.

3. In a mixing bowl, combine the milk, flour, mustard, black pepper and salt. Set aside.

4. Over medium stove flame, heat the oil in a skillet or saucepan (preferably of medium size).

5. Sauté the garlic until softened and fragrant, stirring in between.

6. Add the milk mixture and let it simmer. Add the tarragon, lemon juice and lemon zest; mix to combine.

7. Add the cooked pasta, asparagus, and simmer until the sauce thickens, stirring frequently.

8. Top with parmesan cheese and serve warm.

Nutrition: Calories – 402|Fat – 31g|Carbs – 33g|Fiber – 6g|Protein – 44g

Mussels Linguine Delight

Preparation Time: 20 minutes

Cooking Time: 10 minutes

Servings: 4

Ingredients:

- 1 lb. mussels, cleaned and debearded
- 1 tbsp. olive oil
- ½ tsp. oregano
- ½ tsp. basil, chopped
- 1 clove garlic, minced
- 1 lemon, wedges
- 8 oz. whole-wheat linguine pasta
- 1 pinch pepper flakes, crushed
- 1 (14.5 oz.) can tomatoes, crushed
- ¼ cup white wine

Directions:

1. Pour the water into a deep saucepan and boil it. Add the pasta and some salt; cook it as per

package directions. Drain the water and set aside the pasta.

2.   Over a medium stove flame; heat the oil in a skillet or saucepan (preferably medium size).

3.   Sauté the garlic until softened and fragrant, stir in between.

4.   Add the tomatoes, basil, pepper flakes and oregano. Reduce the heat and simmer the mix.

5.   Add the mussels, wine and increase the heat. Cook for 3-5 minutes.

6.   Wait for the mussels to cook and open. Mix in the pasta.

7.   Garnish with the parsley; serve with some lemon wedges on the side.

Nutrition: Calories – 634|Fat – 15g|Carbs – 36g|Fiber – 7g|Protein – 39g

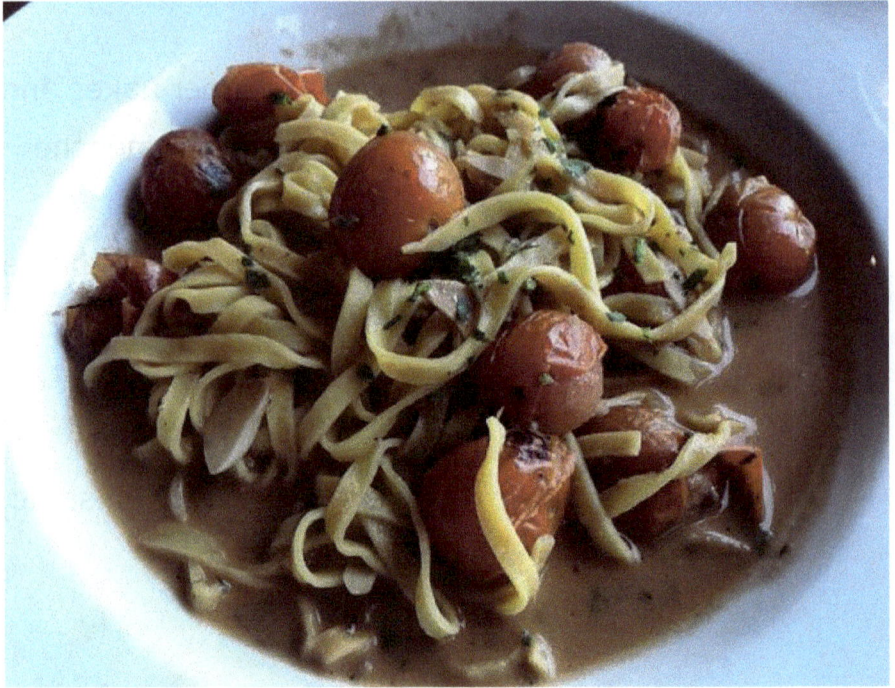

Arugula Pasta Soup

Preparation Time: 15 minutes

Cooking Time: 5 minutes

Servings: 6

Ingredients:

- 7 oz. chickpeas, rinsed
- 4 eggs, lightly beaten
- 2 tbsp. lemon juice
- 3 cups arugula, chopped
- 6 tbsp. parmesan cheese
- 6 cups chicken broth
- 1 pinch of nutmeg
- 1 bunch scallions, sliced (greens and whites sliced separately)
- 1 1/3 cups whole-wheat pasta shells
- 2 cups water
- Ground black pepper, to taste

Directions:

1. In a cooking pot or deep saucepan, combine the pasta, scallion whites, chickpeas, water, broth and nutmeg.
2. Heat the mixture; cover and bring to a boil.
3. Take off the lid and simmer the mixture for about 4 minutes. Add the arugula and cook until it is wilted.
4. Mix in the eggs and season with black pepper and salt.
5. Mix in the lemon juice and scallion greens. Top with the parmesan cheese; serve warm.

Nutrition: Calories – 317|Fat – 7g|Carbs – 32g|Fiber – 6g|Protein – 38g

Pasta with garlic and Hoat Pepper

Preparation Time: 25 minutes

Cooking Time: 4 minutes

Servings: 4

Ingredients:

- 400g Spaghetti
- 8 tbsp. Extra virgin olive oil
- 4 cloves garlic, chopped
- 1 Chili pepper
- Coarse salt

Directions:

1. Put the water to boil, when it comes to a boil add salt and dip the spaghetti.
2. Meanwhile, in a saucepan heat the oil with the garlic deprived of the inner and chopped germ and the chopped peppers. Be careful: the flame should be sweet and the garlic should not darken.
3. Halfway through cooking, remove the spaghetti and continue cooking in the pan with

the oil and garlic, adding the cooking water as if it were a risotto.

4.   When cooked, serve the spaghetti.

Nutrition: Calories 201, Fat 4.3g, Protein 5.8g, Carbs 20.1g

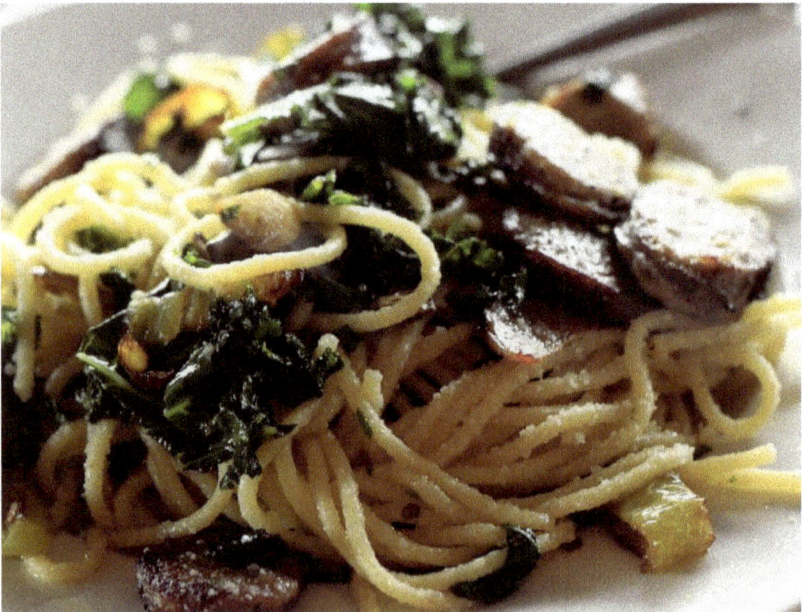

Stuffed Pasta Shells

Preparation Time: 15 minutes

Cooking Time: 10 minutes

Servings: 4

Ingredients:

- 5 Cups Marinara Sauce
- 15 Oz. Ricotta Cheese
- 1 ½ Cups Mozzarella Cheese, Grated
- ¾ Cup Parmesan Cheese, Grated
- 2 tbsp. Parsley, Fresh & Chopped
- ¼ Cup Basil Leaves, Fresh & Chopped
- 8 Oz. Spinach, Fresh & Chopped
- ½ tsp. Thyme
- Sea Salt & Black Pepper to Taste
- 1 lb. Ground Beef
- 1 Cup Onions, Chopped
- 4 Cloves Garlic, Diced
- 2 tbsp. Olive Oil, Divided
- 12 Oz. Jumbo Pasta Shells

Directions:

1. Start by cooking your pasta shells by following your package instructions. Once they're cooked, then set them to the side.

2. Press sauté and then add in half of your olive oil. Cook your garlic and onions, which should take about four minutes. Your onions should be tender, and your garlic should be fragrant.
3. Add your ground beef in, seasoning it with thyme, salt, and pepper, cooking for another four minutes.
4. Add in your basil, parsley, spinach and marinara sauce.
5. Cover your pot, and cook for five minutes on low pressure.
6. Use a quick release, and top with cheeses.
7. Press sauté again, making sure that it stays warm until your cheese melts.
8. Take a tbsp. of the mixture, stuffing it into your pasta shells.
9. Top with your remaining sauce before serving warm.

Nutrition: Calories: 710, Protein: 45.2 g, Fat: 23.1 g, Carbs: 70 g

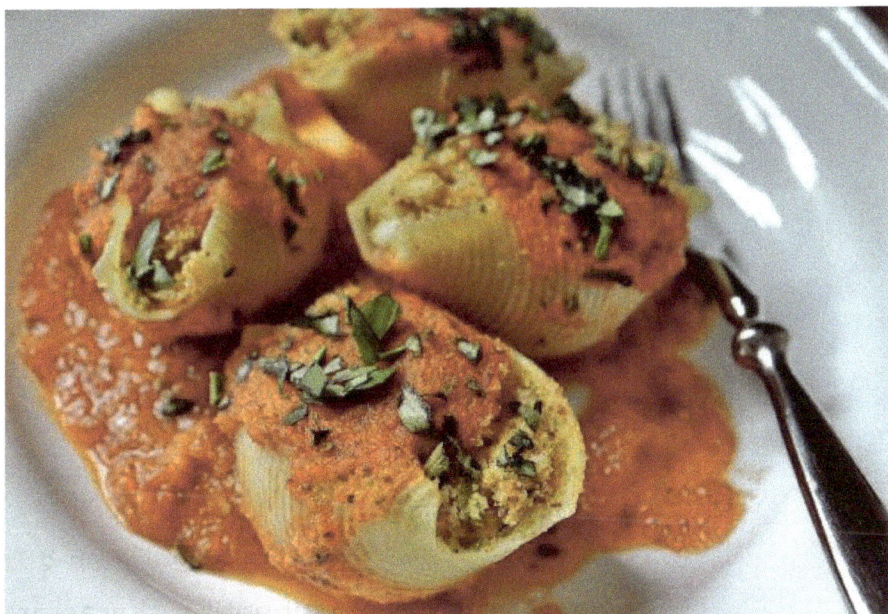

Homemade Pasta Bolognese

Preparation Time: 20 minutes

Cooking Time: 10 minutes

Servings: 4

Ingredients :

- Minced meat 17 oz.
- Pasta 12 oz.
- Sweet red onion1 piece
- Garlic 2 cloves
- Vegetable oil 1 tbsp.
- Tomato paste 3 tbsp.
- Grated Parmesan Cheese 2 oz.
- Bacon3 pieces

Directions:

1. Fry finely chopped onions and garlic in a frying pan in vegetable oil until a characteristic smell.

2. Add minced meat and chopped bacon to the pan. Constantly break the lumps with a spatula and mix so that the minced meat is crumbly.

3. When the mince is ready, add tomato paste, grated Parmesan to the pan, mix, reduce heat and leave to simmer.
4. At this time, boil the pasta. I don't salt water, because for me tomato paste and sauce as a whole turn out to be quite salty.
5. When the pasta is ready, discard it in a colander, arrange it on plates, add meat sauce with tomato paste on top of each serving.

Nutrition: Calories: 1091, Fat: 54.7g, Carbs: 92.8g, Protein: 74g

Asparagus Pasta

Preparation Time: 10 minutes

Cooking Time: 25 Minutes

Servings: 6

Ingredients :

- 8 Oz. Farfalle Pasta, Uncooked
- 1 ½ Cups Asparagus, Fresh, Trimmed & Chopped into 1 Inch Pieces
- 1 Pint Grape Tomatoes, Halved
- 2 tbsp. Olive Oil
- Sea Salt & Black Pepper to Taste
- 2 Cups Mozzarella, Fresh & Drained
- 1/3 Cup Basil Leaves, Fresh & Torn
- 2 tbsp. Balsamic Vinegar

Directions:

1. Start by heating the oven to 400°F, and then get out a stockpot. Cook your pasta per

package instructions, and reserve ¼ cup of pasta water.

2. Get out a bowl and toss the tomatoes, oil, asparagus, and season with salt and pepper. Spread this mixture on a baking sheet, and bake for fifteen minutes. Stir twice in this time.

3. Remove your vegetables from the oven, and then add the cooked pasta to your baking sheet. Mix with a few tbsp. of pasta water so that your sauce becomes smoother.

4. Mix in your basil and mozzarella, drizzling with balsamic vinegar. Serve warm.

Nutrition:

Calories: 307

Protein: 18 g

Fat: 14 g

Carbs: 33 g

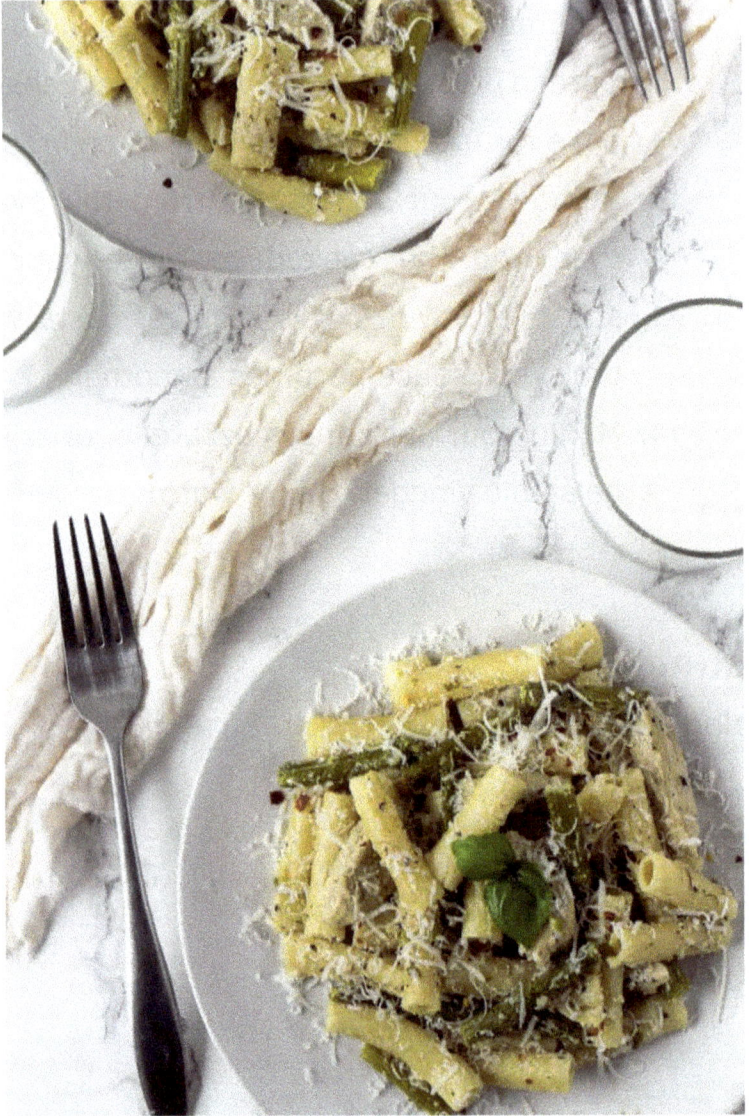

Penne Bolognese Pasta

Preparation Time: 15 minutes

Cooking Time: 20 minutes

Servings: 2

Ingredients :

- Penne pasta 7 oz.
- Beef 5 oz.
- Parmesan Cheese 1 oz.
- Celery Stalk 1 oz.
- Shallots 26 g
- Carrot 1.5 oz.
- Garlic 1 clove
- Thyme 1 g
- Tomatoes in own juice 6 oz.
- Parsley 3 g
- Oregano 1 g
- Butter 20 g
- Dry white wine 50 ml
- Olive oil 40 ml

Directions:

1. Pour the penne into boiling salted water and cook for 9 minutes.
2. Roll the beef through a meat grinder.

3. Dice onion, celery, carrots and garlic in a small cube.
4. Fry the chopped vegetables in a heated frying pan in olive oil with minced meat for 4–5 minutes, salt and pepper.
5. Add oregano to the fried minced meat and vegetables, pour 50 ml of wine, add the tomatoes along with the juice and simmer for 10 minutes until the tomatoes are completely softened.
6. Add the boiled penne and butter to the sauce and simmer for 1-2 minutes, stirring continuously.
7. Put in a plate, sprinkle with grated Parmesan and chopped parsley, decorate with a sprig of thyme and serve.

Nutrition:

Calories: 435

Protein: 18 g

Fat: 14 g

Carbs: 33 g

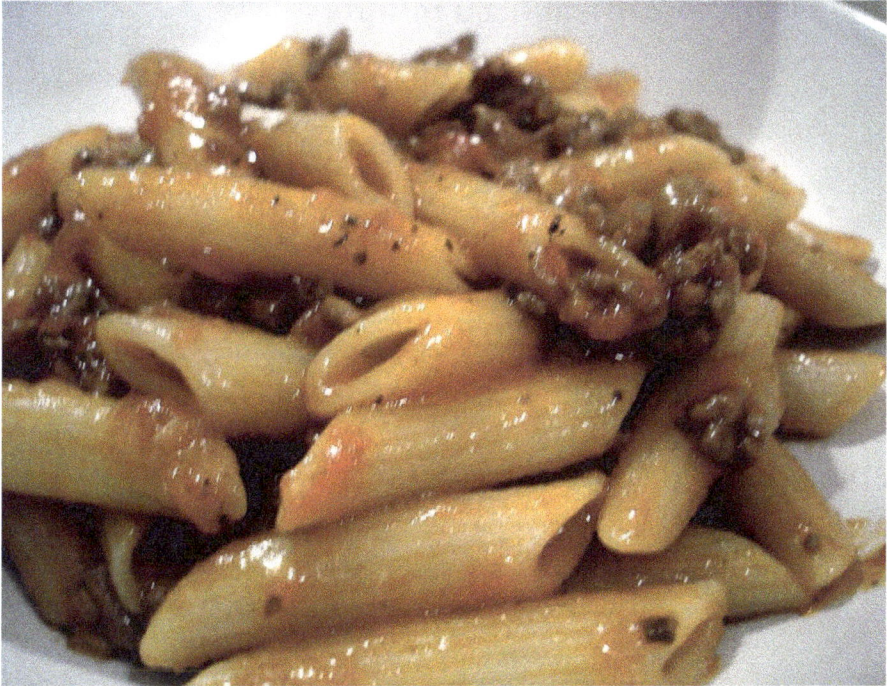

Quick Pasta Bolognese

Preparation Time: 10 minutes

Cooking Time: 25 minutes

Servings: 2

Ingredients :

- Ground beef 17 oz.
- Garlic 2 cloves
- Tomato paste 3 tbsp.
- Tomatoes 14 oz.
- Beef broth 150 ml
- A mixture of Italian herbs 1 tsp.
- Penne pasta 14 oz.
- Basil leaves to taste
- Fresh mushrooms to taste

Directions:

1. Prepare the paste following the instructions on the packaging.

2. Heat the oil in a pan, sauté the minced meat for 5 minutes, then add the mushrooms and fry for another 3 minutes. Add garlic and tomato paste and simmer for 2 minutes. Add tomatoes, broth or wine, dried herbs and spices. Bring to a boil and simmer for 10 minutes.

3. Drain the water from the pasta, mix it with the sauce, sprinkle with basil leaves on top.

Nutrition:

Calories: 710

Protein: 18 g

Fat: 14 g

Carbs: 33 g

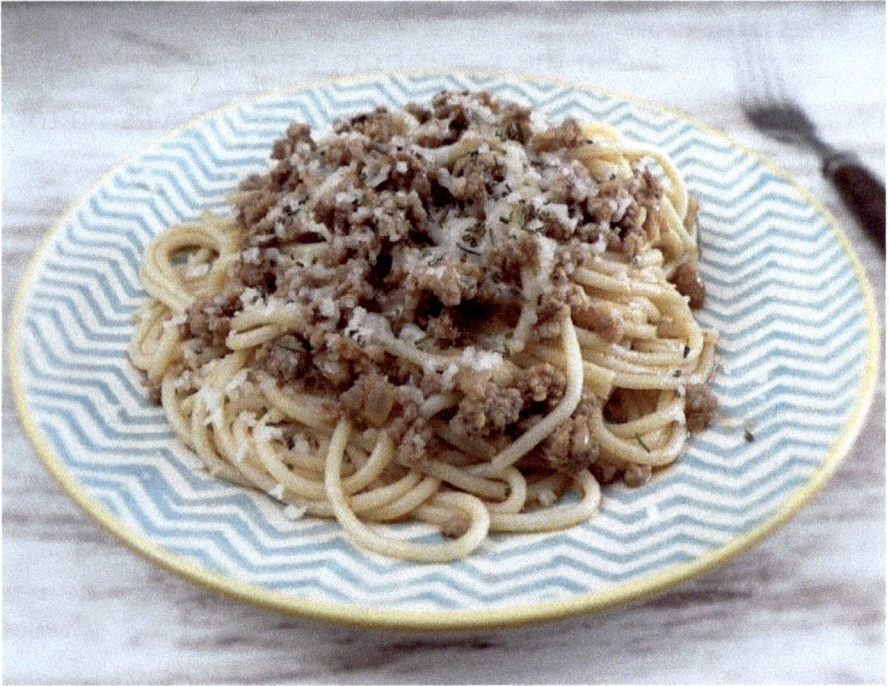

Pilaf with Cream Cheese

Preparation Time: 10 minutes

Time: 30 Minutes

Servings: 4

Ingredients:

- 2 Cups Yellow Long Grain Rice, Parboiled
- 1 Cup Onion
- 4 Green Onions
- 3 tbsp. Butter
- 3 tbsp. Vegetable Broth
- 2 tsp. Cayenne Pepper
- 1 tsp. Paprika
- ½ tsp. Cloves, Minced
- 2 tbsp. Mint Leaves, Fresh & Chopped
- 1 Bunch Fresh Mint Leaves to Garnish
- 1 tbsp. Olive Oil
- Sea Salt & Black Pepper to Taste

Cheese Cream:

- 3 tbsp. Olive Oil
- Sea Salt & Black Pepper to Taste
- 9 Oz. Cream Cheese

Directions:

1. Start by heating your oven to 360°F, and then get out a pan. Heat your butter and olive oil together, and cook your onions and spring onions for two minutes.
2. Add in your salt, pepper, paprika, cloves, vegetable broth, rice and remaining seasoning. Sauté for three minutes.
3. Cover with foil, and bake for another half hour. Allow it to cool.
4. Mix in the cream cheese, cheese, olive oil, salt and pepper. Serve your pilaf garnished with fresh mint leaves.

Nutrition:

Calories: 364g

Protein: 5g

Fat: 30g

Carbs: 20g

Herbed Pasta

Preparation Time: 15 minutes

Cooking Time: 15 minutes

Servings: 4

Ingredients:

- 1 (8-oz.) package linguini pasta
- 2 tbsp. olive oil
- 1 tbsp. garlic, minced
- 1 tbsp. dried oregano, crushed
- 1 tbsp. dried basil, crushed
- 1 tsp. dried thyme, crushed
- 2 cups plum tomatoes, chopped

Directions:

1. In a large pan of lightly salted boiling water, add the pasta and cook for about 8-10 minutes or according to package's directions.
2. Drain the pasta well.

3.   In a large skillet, heat oil over medium heat and sauté the garlic for about 1 minute.
4.   Stir in herbs and sauté for about 1 minute more.
5.   Add the pasta and cook for about 2-3 minutes or until heated completely.
6.   Fold in tomatoes and remove from heat. Serve hot.

Nutrition:

Calories 301

Fat 8.9 g

Carbs 47.7 g

Protein 8.5 g

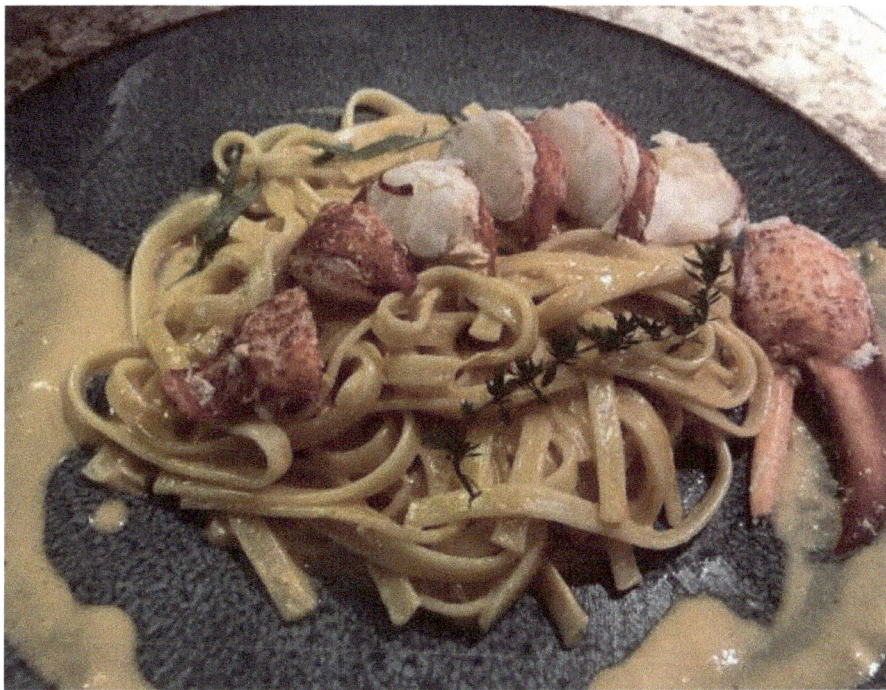

Pasta with Veggies

Preparation Time: 15 minutes

Cooking Time: 20 minutes

Servings: 6

Ingredients:

- 3 tomatoes
- 1-lb. farfalle pasta
- ¼ cup olive oil
- 1-lb. fresh mushrooms, sliced
- 3 garlic cloves, minced
- 1 tsp. dried oregano, crushed
- 1 (2-oz.) can black olives, drained
- ¾ cup feta cheese, crumbled

Directions:

1. In a large pan of the salted boiling water, add the tomatoes and cook for about 1 minute.
2. With a slotted spoon, transfer the tomatoes into a bowl of ice water.
3. In the same pan of the boiling water, add the pasta and cook for about 8-10 minutes.
4. Drain the pasta well.

5. Meanwhile, peel the blanched tomatoes and then chop them.
6. In a large skillet, heat oil over medium heat and sauté the mushrooms and garlic for about 4-5 minutes.
7. Add the tomatoes and oregano and cook for about 3-4 minutes.
8. Divide the pasta onto serving plates and top with mushroom mixture.
9. Garnish with olives and feta and serve.

Nutrition:

Calories 446

Fat 15.1 g

Carbs 62.2 g

Protein 15.2 g

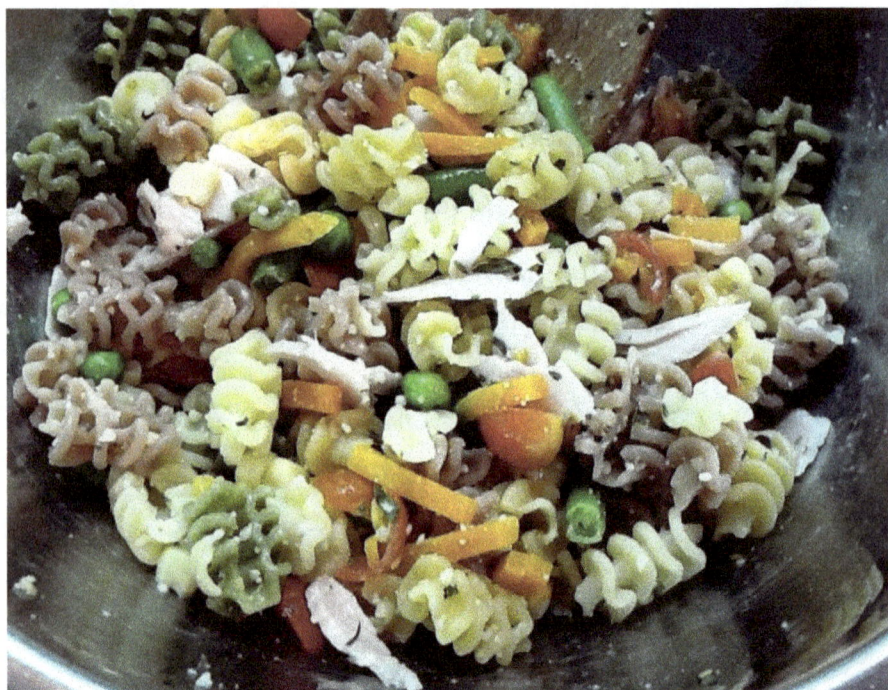

Pasta with Chicken & Veggies

Preparation Time: 15 minutes

Cooking Time: 10 minutes

Servings: 7

Ingredients:

- 3 tbsp. olive oil
- 1-lb. boneless, skinless chicken breast, sliced diagonally
- 1 (8½-oz.) jar sun-dried tomatoes, julienned
- 2 tbsp. garlic, minced
- 1-lb. angel hair pasta
- 1 (8½-oz.) can water-packed artichoke hearts, quartered and drained
- ½ cup kalamata olive, pitted
- ¼ cup fresh basil
- 6 oz. feta cheese, crumbled
- ¼ cup heavy cream
- 1 tsp. dried oregano
- Salt and ground black pepper, as required

Directions:

1. In a skillet, heat the oil over medium heat and sear the chicken strips for about 5-6 minutes or until browned completely.
2. Add the sun-dried tomatoes and garlic and sauté for about 2 minutes.
3. Meanwhile, in a large pan of the salted boiling water, add the pasta and cook for about 5-6 minutes.
4. Drain the pasta well.
5. In the skillet, add the artichoke hearts, olives, basil and feta cheese and sauté for about 1 minute.
6. Add the cream and stir to combine.
7. Stir in the oregano, salt and black pepper and remove from the heat.
8. In a large serving bowl, add the pasta and chicken mixture and toss to coat well.
9. Serve immediately.

Nutrition:

Calories 429

Fat 17.1 g

Carbs 43.1 g

Fiber 2.7 g

Protein 26.3 g

Pasta with Shrimp & Spinach

Preparation Time: 15 minutes

Cooking Time: 10 minutes

Servings: 4

Ingredients:

- 1 cup sour cream
- ½ cup feta cheese, crumbled
- 3 garlic cloves, chopped
- 2 tsp. dried basil, crushed
- ¼ tsp. red pepper flakes, crushed
- 8 oz. fettuccine pasta
- 1 (10-oz.) packages frozen spinach, thawed
- 12 oz. medium shrimp, peeled and deveined
- Salt and ground black pepper, as required

Directions:

1. In a large serving bowl, add the sour cream, feta, garlic, basil, red pepper flakes and salt and mix well.
2. Set aside until using.
3. In a large pan of the lightly salted boiling water, add the fettucine and cook for about 10 minutes or according to the package's directions.

4. After 8 minutes, stir in the spinach and shrimp and cook for about 2 minutes.

5. Drain the pasta mixture well.

6. Add the hot pasta mixture into the bowl of the sour cream mixture and gently, toss to coat.

7. Serve immediately.

Nutrition:

Calories 457

Fat 19.1 g

Carbs 38.9 g

Fiber 1.7 g

Protein 32.5 g

www.ingramcontent.com/pod-product-compliance
Lightning Source LLC
Chambersburg PA
CBHW050757030426
42336CB00012B/1852